Ketogenic Diet

The Ultimate Beginner's Guide for Understanding the Ketogenic Diet And What You Need to Know

Table Of Contents

Introduction

First off, I really want to thank you for downloading this book. The pages in this book were developed through years of experiences that I have gone through, as well as what has proven to work for others I have talked to and researched. I also want to congratulate you for taking the time to understand the Ketogenic Diet and possibly leading a healthier lifestyle.

This short e-book contains proven steps and strategies on how to achieve nutritional ketosis, a state in which the body utilizes the fat reserves for energy, which will help you efficiently shed those pesky extra pounds without fear of the rebound effect. Nutritional ketosis helps you achieve your ideal weight in as fast as 2 to 4 weeks, without the cravings and extreme restriction of calories, which are the primary causes why most people who are on other diets fail to stick with the program.

Discussed in this book are the advantages and side effects, which will help you decide whether to undergo the diet program or not. The benefits outlined here are taken from years of collective experiences and testimonials backed by scientific research. While some people are enjoying the benefits of a low-carbohydrate diet, it is about time that the secret of a high-energy, zero-craving, easy, fast and efficient diet is shared with you and everyone else looking for it.

I can guarantee that you will find this book useful if you make sure to implement what you learn in the following pages. The important thing is that you IMPLEMENT what you learn. A change in diet and lifestyle is not conquered overnight but the important thing to remember, is that it is definitely possible for you to make the change over time. What I am giving you is the information you need to get started and the guidelines you will need to make that journey.

I recommend that you take notes while you are reading the book. This will ensure that you get the most out of the information in here. I want you to feel that you made a purchase that is worth your money and I want you to look over the notes of this book even after you've finished reading it. The notes will help you to pinpoint exactly what you need to implement and by writing things down, you will be able to recall specifics and how to handle certain situations when they arise.

Lastly, remember that everything in this book has been compiled through research, my own experiences, as well as the experiences of others, so feel free to question what you have read in this book. I encourage you to do your own research on the things that you want to look deeper into. There are many myths created by supplement and pharmaceutical companies, especially around exotic diets such as the Ketogenic Diet, mainly because there is profit to be made off of ignorant consumers. You must be aware of what is true and false and that is why I created this book.

The more you understand your own health and body, the better off you'll be. To adopt the Ketogenic Diet for yourself it will take some preparation and planning on your part, but you can do it! So remember to read with confidence and   an   open   mind!

Chapter 1:

The Need to Lose Weight

With an average daily caloric intake of 3,830, a thousand calories more than the average global consumption of 2,800, and with three-quarters of Americans eating fast food at least once a week, it is no wonder why the United States has one of the highest rates of obesity in the world. To top it off, diseases caused by excess weight are leading to nearly 350,000 deaths per year.

Body Fat as a Metabolic Organ

The health risk of being overweight is attributed to the deposit of excess fat cells. For many years, experts understood fat to be cells that stored energy in the form of glycogen. It wasn't until the past 40-60 years, thanks to the results of new studies, that we have found out fat cells are actually hosts to several chemical reactions.

These reactions result in the production of certain proteins that have hormone-like properties, making them resemble a metabolic organ. These chemicals that fat cells produce, affect the body's sense of hunger, the ability for the body to store fat, as well as fat metabolism.

Body fat has always been regarded as a collection of cells which store energy for future use. When we eat, the excess energy we get from food is stored in these cells, which makes them heavier and larger. However, until recently, scientists have found out that fats are more than just cells for energy storage. They have been found to interfere with normal metabolism, messing up the hunger control system and preventing fat metabolism.

Dangers of Excess Weight

The sudden shifts in the availability of food, from its scarcity during the time of the cavemen to its abundance after the improvements in agriculture and technology, have not given evolution enough time to prepare humans for prolonged and sustained abundance. The programming of our bodies is still centered upon a survival mechanism based on food scarcity. If we were to be likened to machines, it would be like having advanced hardware with an outdated operating system.

The homeostatic operation of our bodies is directed towards saving and storing energy in the hopes of ensuring survival under low-food conditions. This mode of operation, coupled with the instinct to gorge on food whenever available, against easy access to abundant food, has led the present generation towards the perilous path of obesity.

Experts agree that, while excess weight brought about by the storage of energy in the form of fat ensures a person's survival against famine, having tremendous amounts of fat cells for a prolonged period of time has the following negative effects:

Depression

Weight and depression are inseparable, according to a study published in 2010 (Archives of General Psychiatry). Additionally, a review of fifteen studies show that people gain weight because of depression and consequently become depressed because of the new weight gain.

Here are the reasons for it:

Excess weight changes brain chemistry.

Hosting a myriad of fat cells for too long exposes a person to the metabolic effects of the protein they produce. Over time, the interference these fat cells cause, like inducing hunger and preventing fat metabolism, alters the brain chemistry. This imbalance in the neurotransmitters of the brain, of which most, regulate emotions and the perception of optimism, can result in depression.

Society sees overweight people as ugly.

Social responses are powerful external stimuli, which affect how we feel towards ourselves and how we deal with people and everyday situations. In our modern culture, thin is perceived as beautiful. This concept tends to, but not always, lower the self-esteem of those who are overweight, which is known to trigger depression.

Erratic eating patterns cause depression.

Our circadian rhythm does not only regulate our sleeping patterns. In a way, it tells us something about the cycle of the chemical processes that happen inside of our body. Because of this, our body operates with the expectation that it will get energy at certain times of the day and expend the said energy at other times. When this rhythm is disrupted, our body responds through our emotions. Studies reveal odd eating patterns, eating disorders, and the physical discomfort caused by being obese, can result in depression.

Medications for depression contribute to weight gain.

Experts say that almost all people under antidepressant medication, particularly those under Selective Serotonin Reuptake Inhibitors (SSRIs) like Paxil, Zoloft, Prozac and Lexapro, tend to gain weight much easier than the average person. A review published in 2003 showed that this side effect of most antidepressant drugs is observed to occur after six months or more of use.

Heart Disease and Stroke

It has been observed that those who carry excess weight also tend to have high blood pressure and unhealthy levels of bad cholesterol in the blood. These conditions lead to cardiovascular problems such as heart disease and stroke. Compared to lean people, those who are obese have six times the likelihood of having high blood pressure.

It is known that about 22 pounds of excess weight can lead to a 24% increase in the risk of a stroke. The data provided by the Archives of Internal Medicine, published on 2007, found that being overweight increased a person's risk of heart disease by 32%, and that being obese (grossly overweight) increased the risk to 81%.

Cancer

In a study conducted by the American Cancer Society, in which the data was monitored for 16 years with a group of 900,000 American adults, it was found that overweight women had a 62% increased risk of dying from cancer than those in the normal, healthy weight range. Similarly, overweight men had a 52% increased risk of dying from cancer than those in the healthy weight range.

In a similar but separate study conducted by the National Cancer Institute (NCI) in 2007, it was estimated that about 50,500 (7 percent) of new cases of cancer in women and 34,000 (4 percent) in men were attributed to obesity. Although the percentage of the different types of cancers varied, some types of cancer had up to a 40% chance of occurrence in people who were overweight.

Diabetes

Statistics show that about 9 out of 10 people with type 2 diabetes are obese or overweight. Experts agree that obesity and diabetes are inseparable. In fact, this link has even been formalized by the term "diabesity".

How to Tell if You Need to Lose Weight

The quickest possible way to determine whether one is overweight or not is to take his/her weight and height, and compute the Body Mass Index or BMI. People with a BMI of 25-29 are considered overweight while a BMI of 30 or greater indicates obesity.

There are other signs, as well, that are good indicators of being overweight or obese. These are some signs of being overweight:

You have a big belly.

A good indicator of whether one is in the healthy weight range is the size of the waist. A waist size of more than 40 inches for men and 35 inches for women, usually indicates being overweight.

You have excess food cravings.

Various studies have revealed that overweight people have abnormally fluctuating levels of blood sugar, which affects and interferes with the normal functioning of the region in the brain that regulates impulses. This explains why the craving for high-calorie foods is usually high among overweight individuals.

Chapter 2:

The Low Carbohydrate Diet

Mechanism of Fuel Metabolism from A Ketogenic Diet

Our body acquires energy from the combination of the three macronutrients: carbohydrates, proteins and fats. To use energy under low carbohydrate conditions, our body first turns to its small reserves of carbohydrates, which are quickly depleted. Once these glycogen stores are used up, our body resorts to finding alternatives such as the free fatty acids (FFA), which are utilized by most tissues in the body. Not all organs, however, are able to derive energy from FFA. The brain, for instance, and the nervous system are unable to use FFA for fuel.

The by-product of an incomplete FFA breakdown in the liver, called ketone bodies, are another source of energy, especially for tissues that are unable to use FFA. Large amounts of ketone bodies in the blood produce a metabolic state called ketosis, where the body's usage and production of glucose decreases, as well as the breakdown of protein to be used as an energy source.

Hormonal Aspects

Two hormones are responsible for energy metabolism within the body. One is insulin, which moves nutrients out of the bloodstream and into the tissues. Its primary purpose is energy storage, such as causing glucose to be stored as glycogen and FFA as triglycerides. The other is Glucagon, which stimulates the body to utilize the stored glycogen in the muscles in order to provide glucose for the body.

Under low-carbohydrate conditions, the level of insulin in the bloodstream dips while the level of Glucagon rises, which results in the increased release of FFA from fat cells and accelerated FFA metabolism in the liver. This results in the production of acetone, acetoacetic acid and beta-hydroxybutyric acid, collectively known as ketone bodies, creating ketosis. Additionally, a ketogenic diet affects other hormones, as well, which helps shift fuel usage from carbohydrates to fats.

Physical Activity

Because carbohydrates are very essential in sustaining high intensity physical exercises, people under a ketogenic diet will find it useful to stick to low-intensity exercises. Those who insist on high-intensity physical activities should try suggested modifications with the diet and variants that incorporate minimal amounts of carbohydrates without interrupting ketosis.

Chapter 3:

The Benefits of A Low Carbohydrate Diet

It has been established by dietitians that, although extreme diets have unique advantages to them, they are not perfect and have side effects, of which some are even harmful to the health if not kept in check.

A ketogenic diet suppresses food cravings.

The trouble with most diets is that they make dieters hungry and increase their longing for food. This is the primary reason why most people fail to finish the whole course of a diet and give up along the way. The best feature of the ketogenic diet is that it has the ability to suppress hunger.

While it would be normal to suspect that ketone bodies play a role in hunger suppression (which it does not), what actually helps curb cravings is the limited amount of carbohydrates that a person can take in (800 calories/day). It has been found in numerous studies that by limiting the amount of carbohydrates consumed and by not restricting much in regards to protein and fat, a suppressant effect on a person's cravings for food can take place.

Cutting carbohydrates results in faster weight loss.

Compared to other popular diets, the ketogenic diet offers the fastest weight loss in the first two weeks, as cutting carbohydrates typically results in rapid excess water loss. This is because, as the insulin levels in your blood dips, the kidneys are forced to excrete the excess sodium, which is responsible for maintaining the excess water in the body.

Compared to those who are on low-fat diets, ketogenic dieters are observed to lose 2-3 times as much weight on average, even if those on low-fat diets actively restrict their caloric intake.

A ketogenic diet is effective against visceral fat.

Also known as toxic fat, visceral fats are fat cells that lodge around the vital organs and in the abdominal cavity. Visceral fat formation can be noticed through the formation of a gut or big tummy. For years, experts have correlated visceral fats to increased resistance to insulin, metabolic syndromes and cardiovascular diseases.

Low-carb diets cause a drop in the levels of triglycerides.

Although not all experts agree, there has been some research supporting the fact that elevated levels of triglycerides, which are the main forms of fat, are either produced by the body from sources of energy such as carbohydrates or as the end product of the breakdown of fat. High levels of triglycerides are brought about by consumption of carbohydrates and simple sugars, which are absent or are consumed at controlled and minimal amounts on a ketogenic diet.

Cutting carbohydrates boosts HDL cholesterol levels.

Known to many as "good cholesterol" because of its tendency to scavenge for "bad cholesterol" or LDL cholesterol, HDL or high-density lipoprotein levels in the blood are boosted as a long-term benefit of a ketogenic diet. The consumption of saturated fats, which is a feature of a ketogenic diet, boosts HDL cholesterol levels in the blood. A good HDL to LDL ratio indicates a healthier heart.

Fasting causes a blood sugar and insulin drop.

Increased cell exposure to insulin for an extended period of time has been attributed to the development of insulin resistance. The ketogenic diet, in which the intake of sugar and carbohydrates is restricted, blood sugar, and consequently, insulin levels in the blood, drops dramatically.

Blood pressure goes down.

Although it is not a disease, and some people could have it without sustaining damage or showing symptoms of damage, high blood pressure or hypertension, is a serious medical condition that leads to life-threatening health problems such as coronary heart disease, stroke, kidney failure and heart failure. One of the primary factors from high blood pressure is high levels of sugar in the blood and insulin resistance.

Dietary intervention, in which glucose and insulin metabolism are effectively changed, were found to lower blood pressure significantly. The ketogenic diet affects a person similarly. Sustaining a low-carbohydrate diet helps a person to maintain normal blood pressure.

Ketogenic diets effectively treat metabolic syndrome.

The five factors that can lead to metabolic syndrome are elevated blood pressure, increased levels of blood sugar, abdominal obesity, decreased HDL level and increased LDL level.

These factors are effectively arrested by restricting carbohydrate and sugar intake.

Ketogenic diets are used to treat brain disorders.

It has been known that ketosis effectively prevents seizures in epileptic patients. Experts believe that the change from the body's use of glucose as an energy source to using ketone bodies, creates a chemical change in the brain which can prevent the onset of epileptic attacks. In a study investigating the effect of ketogenic diets on children, it was found that there were 50% fewer seizures when a child was on a ketogenic diet versus a traditional diet. Nearly 15% of the subjects reported not experiencing a seizure at all.

Chapter 4:

Side Effects of A Ketogenic Diet

A low-carbohydrate diet, especially during the first few weeks, while the body is learning to adapt to ketosis, is not completely free of discomfort. While the host of benefits with a ketogenic diet include improvement in over-all health conditions for the dieter, low-carb diets come with a list of side effects that can either interfere with a dieter's resolve to continue with the diet or could affect the health in unexpected ways.

Fatigue

During the first week of being on a ketogenic diet, wherein the blood sugar drops while being replaced by ketones as an energy source, the body will feel fatigued and with less energy. While continuing on the diet, however, as the body gets used to it, fatigue will be replaced by a general feeling of having energy.

Nausea and headaches

In the early stages of weight loss while on a low-carb diet, the body loses a sufficient amount of sodium, which results in excess water loss. This results in an uncomfortable feeling, reminiscent of mild dehydration. This, however, can be avoided by including sodium and potassium in the diet while keeping one's self well-hydrated.

Hypoglycemia and cravings for sugar

As the level of glucagon spikes while on a ketogenic diet, the level of blood insulin, hence the use of glucose as an energy source, drops.

Constipation

Caused by dehydration due to salt loss and magnesium deficiency, another side effect of a ketogenic diet can be constipation. Inclusion of 400 mg of magnesium, cutting back on dairy products, keeping one's self well hydrated, and supplementing with dietary fiber can help counteract this effect.

Muscle cramps

Another effect of losing sodium and electrolytes while on a low-carb diet is muscle cramps. This side effect can be avoided or limited by supplementing with sodium and potassium.

Kidney stones

Because ketone bodies compete with uric acid excretion from the kidneys, in which the latter is given priority, monosodium urate salt crystals can possibly form in the kidneys, a condition commonly referred to as kidney stones. This can be avoided by drinking at least a gallon of water per day while on the diet.

Chapter 5:

Starting, Maintaining And Ending The Diet

Ketosis, the metabolic state that is the goal of the ketogenic diet, occurs in two stages. One is beneficial, called nutritional ketosis, wherein three ketone bodies, namely acetoacetate (AcAc), acetone and beta-hydroxybutyrate (BHB) exist in controlled amounts at a safe ratio.

The other is detrimental and called ketoacidosis, wherein the body fails to regulate the ratio and concentration of the said ketone bodies in the blood, causing physiological stress and discomfort that could even prove fatal if left unchecked. Achievement of nutritional ketosis, also called ketoadaptation, is the primary goal of this diet.

Ketosis and the Three Macronutrients

Because of the use of nutritional ketosis in preventing and treating epileptic seizures since the time of the ancient Greeks, experts have already built, refined and mastered the attainment of this metabolic state. Thus, the best way to achieve ketosis and receive the maximum benefit from it is to refer to what doctors use to treat epilepsy.

Over the years, experts have developed an equation used for planning ketogenic diets for childhood epilepsy. To begin with, experts have grouped foods in categories, namely:

Ketogenic

The attainment of ketosis depends upon the level of glucagon and insulin in the blood. Foods that raise the amount of glucagon in the blood are considered ketogenic and favor the body's attainment of ketosis.

Anti-ketogenic

These are the foods that raise the body's insulin levels and prevent it from attaining ketosis. Macronutrients, which are required by the body, in large and constant supply in order to function well, need to be identified and labeled either ketogenic or anti-ketogenic. This is to be able to determine the exact ratio required by the body to attain ketosis. Here are the macronutrients, plus alcohol, and their effects on ketosis.

Carbohydrates

Since glucose is easily converted to energy within the body, it is the preferred energy source. When carbohydrates are digested, they are converted into and enter the body as glucose, inhibiting ketone body formation, lowering glucagon levels and raising insulin levels in the blood. With this, carbohydrates are considered to be 100% ketogenic.

Protein

A fraction of dietary protein intake (58%) is converted to glucose, resulting in increased insulin levels and inhibited ketogenesis, thus rendering it partly anti-ketogenic because only 42% contribute to ketogenesis. While its pro-ketogenic effect is attributed to its ability to stimulate the release of glucagon, dietary protein must be restricted to a predetermined amount, as too much intake of it could cause an excessive release of glucose in the blood stream, prompting insulin production as a response.

Fat

When metabolized, a glycerol portion of triglycerides, which make up 10% of the total fat grams, is converted into glucose, thus rendering fat 90% ketogenic.

Alcohol

Although alcohol is neither ketogenic nor anti-ketogenic, it is important to include it in this list since excessive intake of it while in ketosis could cause acidosis, which is fatal. It can also limit the ability of the liver to process FFA and interfere unpleasantly with ketosis.

Starting and Maintaining A Low Carbohydrate Diet

Count carbohydrate content of foods.

There are many online and printed resources that can provide you with the macronutrient contents of different food items. This will help you to track the amount of carbohydrates that you take in. The body can survive almost indefinitely without dietary carbohydrates (provided that a person consumes sufficient protein backed by vitamins and minerals to avoid malnutrition).

However, most foods contain carbohydrates and a dieter could consume more than his or her desired amount to initiate and maintain ketosis fairly quickly. A great resource for tracking macronutrient contents online is www.myfitnesspal.com.

Eat with a ratio of 4:1:1.

This is four grams of healthy fats for every gram of protein and carbohydrate. That is, if you consume, for example, 100 grams of carbohydrates (the maximum carbohydrate intake requirement for ketosis to develop), you are advised to consume 100 grams of protein and 400 grams of fat. If you are an athlete that is preforming strength-required activities, you can raise the ratio to 4:2:1, in favor of protein.

Remove carbohydrate sources from your kitchen.

To avoid temptation and to facilitate a change, remove all carbohydrate-rich foods, even complex carbohydrate foods, from your kitchen. Keep only those carbohydrate sources with low carb content.

Stockpile on foods that fit in a Ketogenic Diet.

These include sources of protein, healthy fats and carbohydrates based on the list provided. Prioritize whole and real foods more than processed and packaged "low carb" foods. Great foods that are high in fat include, avocados, almonds, and nut butters.

Plan and cook your meals.

A ketogenic diet is a shift in lifestyle for most people. It does not rely on fast food and quick energy sources. Prompt for quality foods and take time to prepare them for yourself. Careful planning followed by preparation is needed in order to start and sustain the diet.

Keep yourself hydrated.

As mentioned earlier, excess water, which is held on by the body, will be expelled by the kidney at the start of restricting carbohydrate intake. You need to drink a sufficient amount of water in order to keep hydrated as well as to help expel excess uric acid as ketosis tends to cause an increase in uric acid levels in the blood. Drinking water can also help to curb your appetite, as it works to fill you up. Remember, one to two gallons daily is a great amount, especially if you are aiming for fat loss.

Conclusion

I worked hard on creating the best guide for the Ketogenic Diet that I could. These are all the strategies and information that has worked for me, as well as others that I have talked to and researched. I hope this book was able to help you to get a better understanding of the Ketogenic Diet, its origins, benefits, and how to do it safely.

Hopefully it helped you with deciding on whether or not to go on a Ketogenic Diet program and also motivated you to start shedding those extra pounds for a longer and healthier life. You can also share the knowledge outlined in this book to friends and family who are struggling with health issues.

The next step is to put down this book (keep it for reference, though) and weigh out the pros and cons of the Ketogenic Diet for your own situation. If you are interested, check with your doctor and dietician before you get started.

If you feel like you learned something from this book, please take the time to share your thoughts with me by sending me a message. I would also appreciate it if you left a review on Amazon!

Thank you and good luck in your journey!